Metabolic Confusion Diet for Endomorph Women

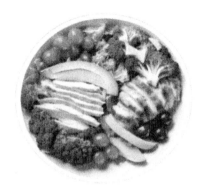

Unlock Your Body's Potential and Achieve Your Ideal Figure

Isabella Hart

WELCOME TO YOUR METABOLIC MAKEOVER, GORGEOUS. IT'S TIME TO FALL IN LOVE WITH YOUR ENDOMORPH SELF!

ISABELLA HART

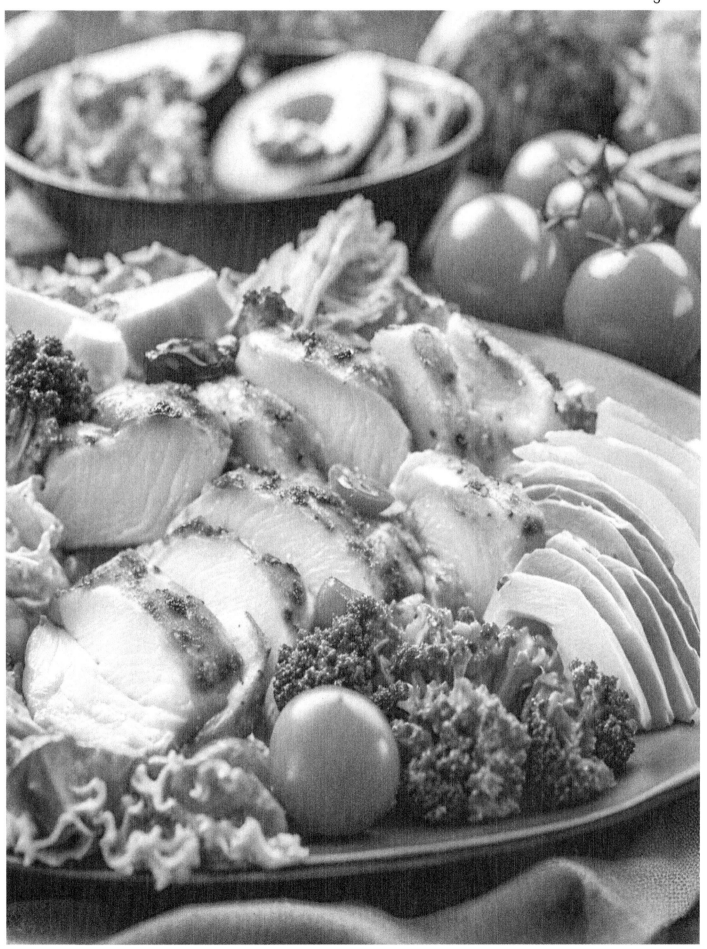

Hey there, **beautiful! Yes, you** -Welcome to your personal **metabolic revolution.** If you've picked up this book, you're probably an endomorph woman who's been on a wild ride with your body. Trust me, I get it. We're like that friend who remembers every detail – except our bodies are holding onto every calorie!

But here's the truth: you're not broken. Your body isn't failing you. It's just playing by its own rules, and it's time we learned to speak its language.

This book is for you – the curvy goddess who's done with one-size-fits-all diets that work for everyone but her. It's for the woman ready to outsmart her genes and find peace with food and her figure.

You're not alone in this journey. There are millions of us out there, all searching for the same answers. And guess what? We're about to crack the code together.

So take a deep breath. Let go of the guilt and frustration. You're about to embark on a journey that'll change how you see food, your body, and yourself.

Ready to confuse your metabolism and show it who's boss? Ready to embrace your curves while working towards your healthiest, happiest self?

Let's do this! Turn the page, and let's start this adventure together. Your body is unique, your journey is your own, but with this book? You've got a friend and guide every step of the way.

Welcome to your metabolic makeover, gorgeous.
It's time to fall in love with your endomorph self!

Table Of Content

Introduction

<u>Embracing Your Endomorph Body Type</u>

Imagine you standing in front of the mirror, eyeing your reflection. Those curves, the softness – they're uniquely you. But for years, you've been told these features are something to battle against. Well, honey, it's time to flip that script!

Being an endomorph isn't a curse – it's your superpower waiting to be unleashed. Let's break it down:

What it means to be an endomorph:

Endomorphs are like that cozy sweater everyone wants to cuddle up in. We're naturally curvy, with a knack for building muscle and, yes, holding onto a bit more padding. Our bodies are incredibly efficient at storing energy – a trait that would've made us the envy of our cave-dwelling ancestors!

But here's the kicker: this body type comes with a metabolism that likes to take things slow and steady. It's not lazy, it's just... cautious. And in today's world of quick-fix diets and one-size-fits-all advice, that can feel like swimming upstream.

Common struggles and misconceptions:
Oh, the things we've heard! "Just eat less and move more." "Cut out all carbs." "You're just not trying hard enough." Sound familiar? These well-meaning but misguided nuggets of advice ignore the beautiful complexity of our endomorph bodies.

The truth is, our bodies respond differently to food and exercise. That salad that keeps your ectomorph friend full for hours? It might leave you rumbling for more in no time. And that high-intensity workout that melts pounds off others? It might leave you feeling drained and reaching for comfort food.

But here's where it gets exciting...

The power of working with your genes, not against them:

Imagine for a moment what could happen if you stopped fighting your body and started collaborating with it. That's where the magic happens!

By understanding your unique endomorph needs, you can craft a lifestyle that not only helps you

reach your ideal figure but also floods your body with health benefits. **We're talking:**
- Balanced blood sugar levels, saying goodbye to those energy crashes
- Reduced inflammation, easing those aches and pains
- Improved heart health, keeping your ticker strong
- Better sleep quality, because who doesn't want to wake up feeling fabulous?
- Enhanced mood and mental clarity, helping you conquer your days with a smile

This isn't just about looking good (though that's a nice perk!). It's about feeling vibrant, energized, and in tune with your body.

Let me share a quick story. I had a client, let's call her Lena. For years, she yo-yo dieted, trying every fad that promised quick results. She'd lose weight, then gain it back, feeling more frustrated each time. When she finally learned to work with her endomorph body, everything changed. Not only did she find a sustainable way to manage her weight, but her chronic headaches disappeared, her skin cleared up, and she had energy to play with her kids without needing a nap afterward.

That's the power of embracing your endomorph nature. It's not just about the number on the scale – it's about unlocking a level of health and vitality you might have thought was out of reach.

So, are you ready to stop fighting and start thriving? To unlock the secrets of your endomorph superpowers? Stick with me, gorgeous. We're about to embark on a journey that will transform not just your body, but your entire relationship with food, fitness, and self-love.

Let's turn that efficiency your body loves into your secret weapon. It's time to outsmart your genes and uncover the vibrant, healthy goddess you've always been. Ready? **Let's go!**

Alright, let's dive into the fascinating world of metabolism and unravel the mystery of metabolic confusion. Buckle up, because we're about to get science-y – but don't worry, I promise to keep it as fun as a girls' night out!

Chapter 2

<u>The Science Behind Metabolic Confusion</u>

Breaking down metabolism basics: Picture your metabolism as the engine room of a grand ocean liner – your body. It's constantly humming, keeping everything running smoothly, whether you're sprinting to catch the bus or snoozing on the couch. But unlike a ship's engine, your metabolism isn't just about burning fuel. It's a complex symphony of chemical processes that keep you alive and kicking.

At its core, metabolism is all about energy – how your body takes in, processes, and uses the fuel from your food. It's not just about burning calories; it's about building new cells, repairing tissues, and keeping all your bodily systems in tip-top shape.

Now, let's break it down into three main components:

1. Basal Metabolic Rate (BMR): This is the energy your body needs just to exist. Breathing, pumping blood, maintaining body temperature – all of this requires energy, even when you're doing absolutely nothing. For most people, BMR accounts for about 60-70% of total daily energy expenditure. It's like the idling engine of your car.

2. Thermic Effect of Food (TEF): Every time you eat, your body has to work to digest, absorb, and process the nutrients. This burns calories too! It's usually about 10% of your total daily energy expenditure. Think of it as the energy needed to refuel your car.

3. Physical Activity: This includes both intentional exercise and non-exercise activity thermogenesis (NEAT) – all the fidgeting, walking, and daily movements you do. It can vary widely from person to person and day to day.

Now, here's where it gets interesting for us endomorphs. Our metabolisms tend to be a bit more... let's say, fuel-efficient. We're great at storing energy (hello, curves!), but not always as great at **burning it off.** It's like having a hybrid car when sometimes you want a gas-guzzling sports car.

But fear not! This is where metabolic confusion comes in to shake things up.

How metabolic confusion works:
Metabolic confusion, also known as calorie cycling, is like being the ultimate DJ for your metabolism. You're mixing up the tracks, keeping your body guessing, and avoiding that metabolic plateau that often comes with traditional diets.

Here's the deal: When you consistently eat the same amount of calories day in and day out, your body gets comfortable. It's like, "Cool, I know exactly how much energy I'm getting, so I'll just adjust to use exactly that much." This is especially true if you're on a low-calorie diet. Your body thinks there's a famine and slows everything down to conserve energy.

But with metabolic confusion, you're constantly switching it up. Some days you eat more, some days you eat less. It's like throwing a surprise party for your metabolism every day!

Let's break it down:

1. High-calorie days: These are days when you eat at or slightly above your maintenance calories. It's like telling your body, "Hey, we've got plenty of fuel here! No need to panic and store everything."

2. Low-calorie days: On these days, you eat below your maintenance calories. But because your body is used to those higher-calorie days, it doesn't immediately go into starvation mode.

This back-and-forth keeps your metabolism on its toes. It prevents that adaptive thermogenesis – the fancy term for when your metabolism slows down in response to dieting.

But it's not just about calories. **Metabolic confusion also involves mixing up your macronutrients (proteins, fats, and carbs) and meal timing.** One day you might have a higher-carb day, the next might be higher in protein. You might eat three larger meals one day, and five smaller meals the next.

All of this variety does a few key things:
- It helps regulate hunger hormones like leptin and ghrelin

- It can improve insulin sensitivity

- It keeps your body burning fat for fuel, even on days when you're eating more

Why it's particularly effective for endomorphs:

Now, my curvy queens, this is where things get really exciting for us endomorphs.

Remember how I said our bodies are super efficient at storing energy? Well, that efficiency can work against us when we try traditional diets. Our bodies are like, "Whoa, calories are being restricted? Better hold onto every last one!" It's this protective mechanism that can make weight loss feel like an uphill battle.

But metabolic confusion? It's like speaking our body's language.

Here's why it works so well for endomorphs:

1. It prevents metabolic adaptation: Our bodies are quick to adapt to calorie restriction. By constantly changing things up, we keep our metabolism guessing and working.

2. It's sustainable: Let's be real – super restrictive diets are miserable, especially for us food-loving endomorphs. Metabolic confusion allows for higher-calorie days, making it much easier to stick with long-term.

3. It works with our insulin sensitivity: Endomorphs often have some degree of insulin resistance. The varied calorie and carb intake of metabolic confusion can help improve insulin sensitivity over time.

4. It preserves muscle mass: Higher-calorie days ensure we're getting enough protein and energy to maintain our natural muscle. More muscle means a higher metabolism!

5. It reduces stress on the body: Chronic calorie restriction can increase cortisol (the stress hormone), which can lead to more belly fat storage. The varied approach of metabolic confusion helps keep stress hormones in check.

6. It allows for social flexibility: We can plan our higher-calorie days around social events or holidays, making this approach fit into real life.

7. It taps into our natural metabolic flexibility: Believe it or not, our bodies are designed to deal with varying food intake. By mimicking more natural eating patterns, we're working with our body's innate wisdom.

Now, I know what you might be thinking. "This sounds great, but is it really scientifically proven?"

While the term **"metabolic confusion"** is relatively new, the principles behind it have been studied extensively. Research has shown that calorie cycling can be more effective for fat loss than continuous calorie restriction, especially in the long term. A study published in the International Journal of Preventive Medicine found that subjects who followed a calorie cycling diet lost more weight and body fat compared to those on a standard calorie-restricted diet.

Moreover, a review in the journal "**Obesity Reviews**" highlighted how varying calorie intake can help prevent the metabolic slowdown often associated with weight loss.

But here's the real kicker – it's not just about weight loss. **This approach has been shown to have numerous health benefits:**
- Improved cardiovascular health markers
- Better blood sugar control
- Reduced inflammation
- Enhanced cognitive function
- Improved mood and reduced risk of depression

It's like a total body tune-up!

Now, before you run off to start your metabolic confusion journey, remember – this isn't about crazy swings in your eating. We're not talking about binge days followed by starvation. It's a controlled, mindful approach to varying your intake.

As with any dietary change, it's always a good idea to chat with your healthcare provider, especially if you have any underlying health conditions.

So, **my gorgeous endomorphs**, are you ready to start confusing your metabolism in the best way possible? To work with your body instead of against it? To find a sustainable, enjoyable way to reach your health goals?

Remember, this journey is about more than just changing your body. It's about understanding it, respecting it, and yes, even outsmarting it a little.

It's about finding a way of eating that feels good, both physically and mentally.

In the next chapters, we'll dive into exactly how to implement this approach, complete with meal plans, recipes, and all the tools you need to become a metabolic confusion maestro. Get ready to remix your metabolism and unlock your body's full potential!

Alright, my lovely **endomorph queens,** it's time to roll up our sleeves and get this metabolic party started! We're about to transform not just your body, but your entire approach to food and wellness. So grab a cup of tea (or coffee, I don't judge), and let's dive into prepping your mind and kitchen for this exciting journey.

Chapter 3

<u>Getting Started</u>

<u>Prepping Your Mind and Kitchen</u>

<u>Mindset Shifts for Success</u>

First things first – let's talk about what's going on upstairs. Your mindset is like the foundation of a house. If it's not solid, everything else is gonna be a bit wobbly. So let's lay down some rock-solid mental groundwork:

1. Ditch the "all or nothing" mentality:

Oh honey, how many times have we fallen into this trap? You know, where you eat one cookie and think, "Well, I've ruined everything, might as well eat the whole box"? It's time to kick that thinking to the curb. Life isn't black and white, and neither is your health journey. Progress, not perfection, is our new mantra.

2. Embrace the power of "yet":

Instead of saying **"I can't lose weight"** or **"I'm not good at cooking healthy meals"**, add a little "yet" to the end. "I haven't found the right approach for me... yet." "I'm still learning to cook nutritious meals... yet." It's amazing how this tiny word can open up a world of possibilities.

3. Redefine your relationship with food:

Food isn't the enemy, folks. It's not a reward or a punishment either. It's fuel, it's nourishment, and yes, it's also one of life's great pleasures. Let's start seeing it as a tool to help us feel our best, rather than something to fear or obsess over.

4. Focus on gains, not losses:

Sure, you might be looking to lose some weight. But let's shift that focus to what you're gaining – energy, strength, confidence, better sleep, clearer skin. These non-scale victories are often way more motivating than any number on a scale.

5. Cultivate patience and self-compassion:Remember, your body didn't change

overnight, and it won't change back overnight either. Be patient with yourself. Treat yourself with the same kindness you'd show a dear friend. This journey is about loving yourself to health, not punishing yourself thin.

6. Embrace the journey, not just the destination:

Yes, you have goals. But the real magic happens in the day-to-day choices, the small victories, the lessons learned along the way. Fall in love with the process, and the results will follow.

7. Adopt a growth mindset:

Every "failure" is just data. If something doesn't work, it's not a reflection of your worth – it's just information you can use to adjust your approach. Get curious instead of critical.

Now, let's get practical and talk about setting up your environment for success. Because let's face it, willpower is like a muscle – it gets tired. So we're going to make it as easy as possible to make healthy choices.

Pantry Makeover Essentials:

Alright, it's time for some pantry tough love. We're not going to do anything drastic like throwing out everything you own (unless you want to, in which case, you go girl!). Instead, we're going to gradually phase out the not-so-great stuff and bring in some nutritional superstars.

Here's what your endomorph-friendly pantry should include:

1. Protein powerhouses:

- Canned fish (tuna, salmon, sardines)

- Beans and lentils (great for fiber too!)
- Protein powder (whey, pea, or hemp)
- Nuts and seeds (almonds, walnuts, chia seeds, flaxseeds)

2. Complex carbs:
- Rolled oats
- Quinoa
- Brown rice
- Sweet potatoes

3. Healthy fats:
- Extra virgin olive oil
- Coconut oil
- Avocados
- Nut butters (almond, cashew, peanut)

4. Flavor boosters:- Herbs and spices (turmeric, cinnamon, garlic powder, etc.)

- Apple cider vinegar

- Dijon mustard

- Hot sauce (check for added sugars)

5. Baking alternatives:

- Almond flour

- Coconut flour

- Stevia or monk fruit sweetener

6. Snack options:

- Air-popped popcorn

- Seaweed snacks

- Beef or turkey jerky (watch the sodium)

- Dark chocolate (70% cocoa or higher)

7. Drinks:- Green tea

- Herbal teas
- Sparkling water

Now, what about the stuff that might not serve your new lifestyle? You don't have to toss it all out immediately. Instead, try this approach:

1. Identify the trigger foods: You know, the ones you can't stop eating once you start. These might need to go, or at least be stored out of sight.

2. Gradually replace refined grains with whole grains: Swap white rice for brown, white pasta for whole wheat or legume-based alternatives.

3. Check for hidden sugars: Many condiments and sauces are loaded with sugar. Look for lower-sugar alternatives or make your own.

4. Downsize the junk food: If you're not ready to give up chips or cookies entirely, buy smaller packages or portion them out into single servings.

Remember, this isn't about deprivation. It's about making your healthy choices easy and your less-healthy choices a bit more inconvenient. You're not banning any foods – you're just setting yourself up for success.

Must-Have Kitchen Tools for Your Journey:
Now for the fun part – kitchen gadgets! These tools will make your metabolic confusion journey not just easier, but way more enjoyable too.

1. A good quality blender: This is your secret weapon for smoothies, soups, and even homemade nut butters. Look for one with at least 600 watts of power.

2. Food processor:

Great for chopping veggies, making cauliflower rice, and whipping up homemade energy balls.

3. Spiralizer:

Turn zucchini into noodles, or make fun veggie ribbons to bulk up your meals.

4. Instant Pot or slow cooker:

These are lifesavers for busy days. Throw in your ingredients in the morning, and come home to a perfectly cooked, healthy meal.

5. Air fryer: Get that crispy texture without all the oil. It's great for everything from veggies to lean proteins.

6. Kitchen scale:

Portion control is key for us endomorphs. A scale helps you get a better handle on serving sizes.

7. Meal prep containers:

Invest in some good quality, microwave-safe containers. They'll make batch cooking and meal prepping a breeze.

8. Cast iron skillet:

These are great for high-heat cooking and add a little iron to your diet too.

9. Steamer basket: An easy way to cook veggies while preserving their nutrients.

10. Immersion blender:
Perfect for pureeing soups right in the pot or making single-serving smoothies.

11. Herb scissors:
These multi-blade scissors make adding fresh herbs to your meals quick and easy.

12. Citrus juicer:
Fresh lemon or lime juice can brighten up so many dishes without adding calories.

13. Water infuser pitcher:
Make staying hydrated more fun by infusing your water with fruits and herbs.

Remember, you don't need to run out and buy all of these at once. Start with the basics and gradually build your collection as you explore new recipes and techniques.

Now, let's talk about setting up your kitchen for success:

1. Keep healthy snacks visible: Put a fruit bowl on the counter, or keep cut veggies at eye level in the fridge.

2. Prep in advance: Spend an hour or two on the weekend washing and chopping veggies, cooking some proteins, and portioning out snacks. It'll make weekday meals so much easier.

3. Make water accessible: Keep a water bottle on your desk or nightstand to remind you to stay hydrated.

4. Create a smoothie station: Keep your blender, protein powder, and favorite add-ins all in one spot for easy morning smoothies.

5. Use the "one in, one out" rule: When you bring in new, healthier items, let go of one less healthy item to keep your kitchen from getting cluttered.

6. Keep measuring tools handy: Having measuring cups and spoons easily accessible makes it more likely you'll use them.

7. Make your kitchen a pleasant place to be: Good lighting, some plants, maybe a little music – make your kitchen somewhere you actually want to spend time.

Remember, beautiful, this journey is about progress, not perfection. You don't need to overhaul your entire life overnight. Start with one or two changes and build from there. Celebrate each small victory – the first time you reach for a healthy snack instead of chips, or when you realize you actually enjoy drinking water now.

You're not just changing your diet; you're changing your lifestyle. And that takes time. Be patient with yourself, stay curious, and remember why you started this journey in the first place.

You've got this, my endomorph queen. Your metabolism won't know what hit it! Now, who's ready to start cooking up some delicious, body-loving meals? Let's go!

Chapter 4

The Metabolic Confusion Diet Plan

Alright, my lovely endomorph queens, it's time to get down to the nitty-gritty of the Metabolic Confusion Diet Plan. Grab your favorite mug, fill it with something warm and delicious, and let's dive into the juicy details that will have your metabolism doing the cha-cha in no time!

I hope you're enjoying the book so far! If you find it valuable, I'd greatly appreciate it if you could leave a review once you're finished. Your feedback helps others discover the book and ensures it reaches those who could benefit from it. Thank you for your support!

Structuring Your Eating Schedule: First things first – let's talk about when you're going to eat.

Now, I know what you're thinking: **"Isn't it just breakfast, lunch, and dinner?"** Oh honey, we're about to shake things up in the best way possible!

The key to metabolic confusion is variety, and that includes your eating schedule. We're going to play around with two main approaches:

1. The 5:2 Method:

This isn't about fasting, so don't panic! For five days of the week, you'll eat at your regular calorie level (we'll get to figuring that out soon). Then, for two non-consecutive days, you'll eat at a lower calorie level. It's like giving your metabolism a little surprise party twice a week!

Example:

- **Monday, Tuesday, Thursday, Friday, Sunday:** Regular calorie days

- **Wednesday, Saturday:** Lower calorie days

2. The Zigzag Method:

This is where we really keep your body guessing. You'll alternate between higher and lower calorie days throughout the week. It's like a metabolic rollercoaster (but way more fun and less scary)!

Example:
- **Monday:** Higher calorie
- **Tuesday:** Lower calorie
- **Wednesday:** Higher calorie
- **Thursday:** Lower calorie
- **Friday:** Higher calorie
- **Saturday:** Lower calorie
- **Sunday:** Higher calorie

Now, within these days, we're also going to play around with meal timing. Some days you might do three larger meals, other days you might do five or six smaller meals. The goal is to keep your metabolism on its toes!

Remember, this isn't about starving yourself on the lower calorie days. We're just creating a calorie deficit that's enough to spark your body into fat-burning mode without sending it into starvation panic.

Balancing Macronutrients:

Okay, now let's talk about what's going on your plate. As endomorphs, we need to pay special attention to our macronutrient balance. But don't worry, I promise it's not as complicated as it sounds!

Your macronutrient ratio is going to look something like this:

- **Protein:** 30-35% of total calories

- **Fat:** 30-35% of total calories

- **Carbohydrates:** 30-40% of total calories

Now, before you start panicking about math, let me break it down for you:

Protein:

As an endomorph, protein is your best friend. It helps build and maintain muscle mass (which boosts your metabolism), and it keeps you feeling full. Aim for about 1 gram of protein per pound of your ideal body weight.

Good sources include:

- Lean meats (chicken, turkey, lean beef)

- Fish (salmon, tuna, tilapia)
- Eggs
- Greek yogurt
- Cottage cheese
- Plant-based options like tofu, tempeh, and legumes

Fat:

Don't fear the fat! Healthy fats are crucial for hormone balance and can actually help you burn fat. Focus on unsaturated fats and omega-3s.

Great options include:

- Avocados
- Nuts and seeds
- Olive oil
- Fatty fish like salmon and sardines
- Chia seeds and flaxseeds

Carbohydrates:

Here's where we need to be a bit more careful. As endomorphs, we tend to be more sensitive to carbs. But that doesn't mean we need to cut them out entirely! Focus on complex, fiber-rich carbs and time them around your workouts.

Good choices include:

- Vegetables (all kinds, but especially leafy greens)
- Berries and other low-sugar fruits
- Quinoa
- Sweet potatoes
- Oats
- Brown rice

Now, here's the fun part — we're going to switch up these ratios on different days too! On your higher calorie days, you might increase your carbs a bit. On lower calorie days, you might bump up the protein and fat while lowering the carbs. It's all part of keeping your metabolism guessing!

Sample Meal Plans for Different Calorie Needs: Alright, let's put this all together with some sample meal plans. Remember, these are just examples – feel free to mix and match based on your preferences and dietary needs.

We'll look at three different calorie levels: 1500 calories (lower calorie day), 1800 calories (moderate day), and 2100 calories (higher calorie day). These are general guidelines – your specific calorie needs may vary based on your height, weight, activity level, and goals.

1500 Calorie Day (Lower Calorie):

Breakfast (300 calories):

- Greek yogurt parfait with berries and a sprinkle of low-sugar granola

Mid-morning snack (150 calories):

- Apple slices with a tablespoon of almond butter

Lunch (400 calories):

- Grilled chicken salad with mixed greens, cucumber, tomatoes, and a light vinaigrette

Afternoon snack (150 calories):

- Carrot sticks with hummus

Dinner (500 calories):

- Baked salmon with roasted broccoli and cauliflower rice

1800 Calorie Day (Moderate):

Breakfast (400 calories):

- Veggie and egg white omelet with whole grain toast

Mid-morning snack (200 calories):

- Small handful of mixed nuts and a piece of fruit

Lunch (500 calories):

- Turkey and avocado wrap with a side salad

Afternoon snack (200 calories):

- Greek yogurt with a drizzle of honey and chia seeds

Dinner (500 calories):- Lean beef stir-fry with mixed vegetables and brown rice

2100 Calorie Day (Higher Calorie):

Breakfast (500 calories):

- Protein smoothie bowl topped with sliced banana and a sprinkle of granola

Mid-morning snack (250 calories):

- Hard-boiled eggs and cherry tomatoes

Lunch (600 calories):

- Grilled chicken breast with quinoa and roasted vegetables

Afternoon snack (250 calories):

- Cottage cheese with sliced peaches and a small handful of almonds

Dinner (500 calories):

- Baked cod with sweet potato wedges and steamed green beans

Now, let's talk about how to make this work in real life:

1. Prep is your friend: Spend some time on the weekend (or whatever day works for you) prepping ingredients. Chop veggies, cook some proteins, make a big batch of quinoa or brown rice. It'll make throwing together meals during the week so much easier.

2. Listen to your body: If you're genuinely hungry, eat! This isn't about starving yourself. The goal is to nourish your body, not punish it.

3. Stay hydrated: Sometimes thirst can masquerade as hunger. Aim for at least 8 glasses of water a day.

4. Don't fear leftovers: Cook once, eat twice (or more!). It's a great way to save time and ensure you always have a healthy meal ready to go.

5. Be flexible: If you're supposed to have a lower calorie day but you get invited to a friend's birthday dinner, don't stress! Swap it with a higher calorie day. The beauty of this plan is its flexibility.

6. Focus on whole foods: While we've talked a lot about calories and macros, remember that the quality of your food matters too. Prioritize whole, minimally processed foods most of the time.

7. Enjoy your food: This isn't a diet of deprivation. Find healthy foods you genuinely enjoy. Experiment with herbs and spices to make your meals delicious.

Remember, beautiful, this is your journey. It might take some time to find the perfect balance for you, and that's okay! Be patient with yourself, stay curious, and don't be afraid to adjust things as you go along.

You're not just changing your diet; you're changing your relationship with food and your body. Celebrate the small victories – the first time you make it through a lower calorie day without feeling deprived, or when you realize you actually prefer your homemade stir-fry to takeout.

You've got this, my endomorph queen. Your metabolism is about to meet its match! Now, who's ready to start confusing their taste buds in the most delicious way possible? Let's get cooking!

Chapter 5: Your 7-Day Jumpstart Plan

Alright, my fabulous endomorph queens, it's time to put all that knowledge into action! We're about to embark on a 7-day adventure that'll kickstart your metabolic confusion journey. Grab your favorite pen and let's map out a week that'll have your metabolism doing the happy dance!

Day-by-day meal guide:

Day 1 (Higher Calorie Day - 2000 calories):

Breakfast (500 cal):

- Protein-packed Green Smoothie Bowl

 Recipe: Blend 1 scoop vanilla protein powder, 1 cup spinach, 1/2 frozen banana, 1/2 cup frozen mango, 1 tbsp almond butter, 1 cup almond milk. Top with 1/4 cup low-sugar granola and 1 tbsp chia seeds.

Prep time: 10 minutes

Mid-morning Snack (200 cal):

- 1 medium apple with 2 tbsp natural peanut butter

Lunch (600 cal):

- Grilled Chicken Avocado Salad

  Recipe: 4 oz grilled chicken breast, 2 cups mixed greens, 1/4 avocado, 1/4 cup cherry tomatoes, 2 tbsp feta cheese, 1 tbsp olive oil and balsamic vinegar dressing.

  Prep time: 15 minutes

Afternoon Snack (200 cal):

- 1/2 cup Greek yogurt with 1/4 cup mixed berries and 1 tbsp chopped walnuts

Dinner (500 cal):

- Baked Salmon with Roasted Vegetables

Recipe: 4 oz baked salmon, 1 cup roasted broccoli and cauliflower, 1/2 cup quinoa.

Prep time: 25 minutes, **Cook time:** 20 minutes

Day 2 (Lower Calorie Day - 1500 calories):
Breakfast (300 cal):

- Veggie Egg White Scramble

Recipe: 3 egg whites scrambled with 1/2 cup mixed veggies (spinach, bell peppers, onions), 1 slice whole grain toast.

Prep time: 10 minutes

Mid-morning Snack (150 cal):

- 1 small pear with 1 oz (about 23) almonds

Lunch (400 cal):- Turkey and Hummus Wrap

Recipe: 3 oz sliced turkey, 2 tbsp hummus, lettuce, tomato, cucumber in a whole wheat wrap.

Prep time: 10 minutes

Afternoon Snack (150 cal):

- 1 hard-boiled egg and 1 cup raw carrot sticks

Dinner (500 cal):

- Lean Beef Stir-Fry

Recipe: 3 oz lean beef strips stir-fried with 2 cups mixed vegetables (broccoli, snap peas, carrots) in 1 tsp olive oil, served with 1/3 cup brown rice.

Prep time: 15 minutes, **Cook time: 15** minutes

Day 3 (Moderate Calorie Day - 1800 calories):

Breakfast (400 cal):

- Overnight Oats

Recipe: 1/2 cup rolled oats soaked overnight in 1/2 cup almond milk, mixed with 1 scoop protein powder, 1/2 tbsp chia seeds, 1/2 sliced banana, and a sprinkle of cinnamon.

Prep time: 5 minutes (night before)

Mid-morning Snack (200 cal):

- 1 small apple and 1 oz low-fat cheese

Lunch (500 cal):

- Tuna Nicoise Salad

Recipe: 3 oz canned tuna, 1 hard-boiled egg, 1 cup mixed greens, 5 cherry tomatoes, 5 olives, 2 oz steamed green beans, 1 small boiled potato, 1 tbsp olive oil and lemon dressing.

Prep time: 20 minutes

Afternoon Snack (200 cal):

- 1/4 cup hummus with 1 cup sliced bell peppers

Dinner (500 cal):

- Grilled Chicken with Sweet Potato Mash

Recipe: 4 oz grilled chicken breast, 1/2 medium sweet potato mashed with 1 tsp olive oil, 1 cup steamed broccoli.

Prep time: 10 minutes, Cook time: 25 minutes

Day 4 (Higher Calorie Day - 2000 calories):
Breakfast (500 cal):

- Protein Pancakes

Recipe: Mix 1 scoop protein powder, 1 mashed banana, 1 egg, 1/4 cup oat flour. Cook like regular pancakes. Top with 1 tbsp almond butter and 1/4 cup mixed berries.

Prep time: 15 minutes, **Cook time:** 10 minutes

Mid-morning Snack (200 cal):

- 1 small handful (about 1/4 cup) trail mix (nuts and dried fruit)

Lunch (600 cal):

- Quinoa and Black Bean Bowl

  Recipe: 1/2 cup cooked quinoa, 1/2 cup black beans, 1/4 avocado, 1/4 cup corn, 1/4 cup salsa, 2 tbsp Greek yogurt, over 1 cup mixed greens.

  Prep time: 15 minutes

Afternoon Snack (200 cal):

- 1 small banana with 1 tbsp almond butter

Dinner (500 cal):

- Baked Cod with Roasted Vegetables

Recipe: 4 oz baked cod, 1 cup roasted Mediterranean vegetables (zucchini, eggplant, bell peppers), 1/2 cup brown rice.

Prep time: 15 minutes, **Cook time:** 25 minutes

Day 5 (Lower Calorie Day - 1500 calories):
Breakfast (300 cal):

- Greek Yogurt Parfait

Recipe: 3/4 cup Greek yogurt layered with 1/4 cup mixed berries and 2 tbsp low-sugar granola.

Prep time: 5 minutes

Mid-morning Snack (150 cal):

- 1 medium peach and 1 oz (about 23) almonds

Lunch (400 cal):

- Chicken and Vegetable Soup

Recipe: 3 oz shredded chicken, 1 cup mixed vegetables (carrots, celery, onions), in 1 cup low-sodium chicken broth. Serve with 1 small whole grain roll.

Prep time: 10 minutes, **Cook time:** 20 minutes

Afternoon Snack (150 cal):

- 1/2 cup cottage cheese with 1/2 cup cherry tomatoes

Dinner (500 cal):

- Tofu and Vegetable Stir-Fry

Recipe: 4 oz firm tofu cubes stir-fried with 2 cups mixed vegetables (broccoli, bell peppers, snap peas) in 1 tsp sesame oil, served with 1/3 cup brown rice.

Prep time: 15 minutes, **Cook time:** 15 minutes

Day 6 (Moderate Calorie Day - 1800 calories):

Breakfast (400 cal):

- Veggie and Egg Scramble

   Recipe: 2 whole eggs scrambled with 1/2 cup mixed veggies (spinach, mushrooms, onions), 1 oz low-fat cheese, 1 slice whole grain toast.

   Prep time: 10 minutes, **Cook time:** 10 minutes

Mid-morning Snack (200 cal):

- 1 medium apple with 1 tbsp almond butter

Lunch (500 cal):

- Turkey and Avocado Wrap

   Recipe: 3 oz sliced turkey, 1/4 avocado, lettuce, tomato in a whole wheat wrap. Serve with 1 cup raw vegetable sticks.

   Prep time: 10 minutes

Afternoon Snack (200 cal):

- 1 hard-boiled egg and 1 small handful (about 1/4 cup) baby carrots

Dinner (500 cal):

- Grilled Shrimp Skewers with Quinoa Salad

  Recipe: 4 oz grilled shrimp, 1/2 cup cooked quinoa mixed with 1 cup roasted vegetables (zucchini, bell peppers, cherry tomatoes), 1 tbsp olive oil and lemon dressing.

  Prep time: 20 minutes, **Cook time:** 15 minutes

Day 7 (Higher Calorie Day - 2000 calories):

Breakfast (500 cal):

- Breakfast Burrito

Recipe: 2 scrambled eggs, 1/4 cup black beans, 1/4 avocado, 2 tbsp salsa in a whole wheat tortilla. Serve with 1 small orange.

Prep time: 15 minutes, **Cook time:** 10 minutes

Mid-morning Snack (200 cal):

- 1 small banana and 1 tbsp natural peanut butter

Lunch (600 cal):

- Grilled Chicken Pesto Salad

Recipe: 4 oz grilled chicken breast, 2 cups mixed greens, 1/4 cup cherry tomatoes, 2 tbsp feta cheese, 1 tbsp pine nuts, 1 tbsp pesto dressing.

Prep time: 15 minutes, **Cook time**: 15 minutes

Afternoon Snack (200 cal):

- 1/2 cup Greek yogurt with 1/4 cup mixed berries and 1 tbsp chopped walnuts

Dinner (500 cal):

- Baked Salmon with Roasted Sweet Potato

   Recipe: 4 oz baked salmon, 1 small roasted sweet potato, 1 cup steamed green beans.

   Prep time: 10 minutes, **Cook time:** 25 minutes

Shopping list for the week:

Proteins:

- Chicken breast
- Lean beef
- Salmon
- Cod
- Shrimp
- Turkey slices
- Tofu
- Eggs
- Greek yogurt

- Cottage cheese

- Protein powder

Fruits and Vegetables:

- Spinach

- Mixed greens

- Broccoli

- Cauliflower

- Bell peppers

- Cherry tomatoes

- Cucumbers

- Carrots

- Celery

- Onions

- Zucchini

- Eggplant

- Green beans

- Bananas

- Apples

- Pears

- Peaches

- Mixed berries

- Lemons

Grains and Legumes:

- Quinoa

- Brown rice

- Rolled oats

- Whole grain bread

- Whole wheat wraps

- Black beans

Nuts and Seeds:

- Almonds

- Walnuts

- Chia seeds

- Pine nuts

Dairy and Alternatives:

- Almond milk

- Low-fat cheese

- Feta cheese

Oils and Condiments:

- Olive oil

- Sesame oil

- Balsamic vinegar

- Pesto

- Salsa

- Hummus

Prep tips to stay on track:

1. Sunday Prep Day: Spend a couple of hours on Sunday (or your least busy day) to prep for the week ahead:

- Chop vegetables for easy grab-and-go snacks and quick meal assembly
- Cook a batch of quinoa and brown rice
- Grill or bake chicken breasts for easy protein additions
- Hard-boil a dozen eggs for quick snacks or salad toppers

2. Portion Control: Use small containers to pre-portion snacks and ingredients. This makes it easy to grab the right amount without overthinking it.

3. Salad in a Jar: Prep salads for the week in mason jars. Layer dressing on the bottom, followed by harder veggies, proteins, and greens on top. This keeps everything fresh and crisp.

4. Smoothie Packs: Prepare smoothie ingredients in individual freezer bags. In the morning, just dump the contents in the blender, add liquid, and blend!

5. Overnight Oats: Prepare a few jars of overnight oats at the beginning of the week for quick, grab-and-go breakfasts.

6. Use Your Slow Cooker: Prep ingredients for a slow cooker meal the night before. In the morning, just turn it on and come home to a ready-made dinner.

7. Double Up: When cooking dinner, make extra to use for lunch the next day or to freeze for future meals.

How to adjust portions for your needs: Remember, the calorie levels provided in this plan are just examples. Your specific needs may vary based on your height, weight, activity level, and goals. Here's how to adjust:

1. Calculate your Total Daily Energy Expenditure (TDEE): Use an online calculator to estimate how many calories you burn in a day.

2. Set your goals: For weight loss, aim for a deficit of 300-500 calories per day. For maintenance, eat at your TDEE.

3. Adjust portion sizes: If you need more calories, increase portion sizes or add an extra snack. If you need fewer, reduce portions slightly or skip a snack.

4. Listen to your body: If you're consistently hungry, you may need to increase your intake. If you're always full, you might be eating too much.

5. Focus on nutrient density: When increasing portions, focus on adding more vegetables and lean proteins rather than calorie-dense foods.

6. Be patient and consistent: Give your body time to adjust to the new eating pattern. Consistency is key!

7. Track your progress: Keep a food diary and note how you feel. This can help you fine-tune your portions over time.

Remember, my lovely endomorphs, this plan is a starting point. Feel free to swap meals around based on your preferences or schedule. The key is to keep your body guessing with those calorie and macro shifts while fueling it with nutritious, delicious foods.

You've got this! Your metabolism is about to get the wake-up call of a lifetime. Here's to a week of delicious meals, new cooking adventures, and the start of your metabolic confusion journey. Let's make some magic happen in the kitchen and beyond!

Chapter 6: Breakfast Recipes to Jump-Start Your Metabolism

Rise and shine, my beautiful endomorph queens! It's time to talk about the most important meal of the day - breakfast! We're about to dive into a world of delicious, metabolism-boosting morning meals that'll have you jumping out of bed faster than you can say **"metabolic confusion."**

Now, I know what some of you might be thinking: "But I'm not a breakfast person!" Well, buckle up buttercup, because we're about to change that! Eating a balanced breakfast is crucial for us endomorphs. It kickstarts our metabolism, helps regulate our blood sugar, and sets us up for a day of successful eating. Plus, these recipes are so good, you might just start setting your alarm a little earlier!

Let's break this down into three categories: quick morning fuel options for those busy weekdays, indulgent **(but still healthy!)** weekend brunch ideas, and meal prep solutions for the planning pros among us.

Quick Morning Fuel Options:

1. Power-Packed Green Smoothie

Prep Time: 5 minutes

Ingredients:

- 1 cup unsweetened almond milk

- 1 scoop vanilla protein powder

- 1 cup spinach

- 1/2 frozen banana

- 1 tbsp almond butter

- 1/2 tsp cinnamon

- Ice cubes

Instructions:
Blend all ingredients until smooth. Pour into a glass and enjoy!

Nutritional Value: 300 calories, 20g protein, 30g carbs, 12g fat

Why it works: This smoothie is a nutritional powerhouse. The protein powder and almond butter provide satiating protein and healthy fats, while the spinach offers a dose of vitamins and minerals. The banana adds natural sweetness and potassium, which is great for muscle function.

2. Avocado Toast with Egg

Prep Time: 10 minutes

Ingredients:

- 1 slice whole grain bread

- 1/4 ripe avocado

- 1 large egg

- Salt and pepper to taste

- Red pepper flakes (optional)

Instructions:

1. Toast the bread.

2. Mash the avocado and spread on toast.

3. In a small non-stick pan, fry the egg to your liking.

4. Place the egg on the avocado toast.

5. Season with salt, pepper, and red pepper flakes if desired.

Nutritional Value: 250 calories, 13g protein, 20g carbs, 15g fat

Why it works: This balanced breakfast provides complex carbs from the whole grain bread, healthy fats from the avocado, and protein from the egg. It's a perfect combo to keep you full and focused all morning.

3. Greek Yogurt Parfait

Prep Time: 5 minutes

Ingredients:

- 1 cup Greek yogurt
- 1/4 cup mixed berries
- 1 tbsp chia seeds
- 1 tbsp chopped nuts (almonds or walnuts)
- 1 tsp honey (optional)

Instructions:

Layer all ingredients in a glass or jar. That's it!

Nutritional Value: 300 calories, 25g protein, 25g carbs, 12g fat

Why it works: Greek yogurt is a protein powerhouse, which helps build and maintain muscle mass. The berries provide antioxidants and fiber, while the nuts and chia seeds add healthy fats and extra fiber to keep you feeling full.

Weekend Brunch Ideas:

1. Spinach and Feta Frittata

Prep Time: 10 minutes

Cook Time: 20 minutes

Serves: 4

Ingredients:

- 8 large eggs
- 1/4 cup milk

- 2 cups fresh spinach

- 1/2 cup crumbled feta cheese

- 1/4 cup diced red bell pepper

- 1 tbsp olive oil

- Salt and pepper to taste

Instructions:

1. Preheat oven to 375°F (190°C).

2. In a large bowl, whisk together eggs and milk. Season with salt and pepper.

3. Heat olive oil in an oven-safe skillet over medium heat. Add spinach and bell pepper, cook until spinach is wilted.

4. Pour egg mixture over vegetables. Sprinkle feta on top.

5. Transfer skillet to oven and bake for 15-20 minutes until set and lightly golden.

Nutritional Value (per serving): 250 calories, 20g protein, 5g carbs, 18g fat

Why it works: This frittata is protein-rich thanks to the eggs and feta, which helps preserve muscle mass during weight loss. The vegetables add fiber and nutrients, making this a well-rounded meal that'll keep you satisfied for hours.

2. Protein Pancakes with Berry Compote

Prep Time: 15 minutes

Cook Time: 15 minutes

Serves: 2

Ingredients:

For pancakes:- 1 cup rolled oats

- 2 scoops vanilla protein powder

- 2 ripe bananas

- 2 eggs

- 1/4 cup almond milk

- 1 tsp baking powder

- 1 tsp vanilla extract

For berry compote:

- 1 cup mixed berries (fresh or frozen)

- 1 tbsp water

- 1 tsp honey (optional)

Instructions:

1. Blend all pancake ingredients until smooth.

2. Heat a non-stick pan over medium heat. Pour 1/4 cup batter for each pancake.

3. Cook for 2-3 minutes each side until golden.

4. For compote, simmer berries, water, and honey in a small saucepan for 5-10 minutes until berries break down.

5. Serve pancakes topped with berry compote.

Nutritional Value (per serving): 400 calories, 30g protein, 50g carbs, 10g fat

Why it works: These pancakes are a protein-packed twist on a breakfast favorite. The oats provide complex carbs for sustained energy, while the berries in the compote add antioxidants and natural sweetness without excess sugar.

Meal Prep Breakfast Solutions:

1. Overnight Oats (5 servings)

Prep Time: 15 minutes (plus overnight soaking)

Ingredients (for each serving):

- 1/2 cup rolled oats
- 1/2 cup unsweetened almond milk
- 1/4 cup Greek yogurt

- 1 tbsp chia seeds

- 1 tsp honey

- 1/4 cup mixed berries

Instructions:

1. In 5 jars, combine oats, almond milk, yogurt, chia seeds, and honey.

2. Stir well, cover, and refrigerate overnight.

3. In the morning, top with berries and enjoy!

Nutritional Value (per serving): 250 calories, 15g protein, 35g carbs, 8g fat

Why it works: Overnight oats are a perfect grab-and-go breakfast. The combination of oats and chia seeds provides fiber to keep you full, while the Greek yogurt adds protein. The slow-digesting carbs from the oats provide steady energy throughout the morning.

2. Egg Muffins (12 muffins)

Prep Time: 15 minutes
Cook Time: 20 minutes

Ingredients:

- 12 large eggs
- 1/4 cup milk
- 1 cup chopped mixed vegetables (spinach, bell peppers, onions)
- 1/2 cup shredded cheese
- Salt and pepper to taste

Instructions:

1. Preheat oven to 375°F (190°C). Grease a 12-cup muffin tin.

2. Whisk eggs and milk in a large bowl. Season with salt and pepper.

3. Divide vegetables and cheese among muffin cups.

4. Pour egg mixture over vegetables, filling each cup about 3/4 full.

5. Bake for 20 minutes until set and lightly golden.

6. Cool, then store in an airtight container in the fridge for up to 5 days.

Nutritional Value (per muffin): 90 calories, 8g protein, 2g carbs, 6g fat

Why it works: These portable egg muffins are perfect for busy mornings. They're high in protein, which helps control appetite and preserve muscle mass. The vegetables add fiber and nutrients, making these a balanced breakfast option.

3. Chia Seed Pudding (4 servings)

Prep Time: 10 minutes (plus overnight soaking)

Ingredients:

- 1/2 cup chia seeds

- 2 cups unsweetened almond milk

- 2 tbsp maple syrup

- 1 tsp vanilla extract

- 1/4 cup chopped nuts

- 1 cup mixed berries

Instructions: 1. In a large bowl, whisk together chia seeds, almond milk, maple syrup, and vanilla.

2. Cover and refrigerate overnight.

3. In the morning, stir the pudding and divide into 4 containers.

4. Top with chopped nuts and berries before serving.

Nutritional Value (per serving): 200 calories, 8g protein, 25g carbs, 11g fat

Why it works: Chia seeds are a nutritional powerhouse, packed with fiber, protein, and omega-3 fatty acids. This pudding provides steady energy and helps keep you full throughout the morning.

Remember, my lovely endomorphs, breakfast really is the most important meal of the day for us. It sets the tone for our eating habits and helps rev up our metabolism right from the start. Don't be afraid to mix and match these recipes, or use them as inspiration to create your own metabolic confusion-friendly breakfasts.

The key is to include a balance of protein, healthy fats, and complex carbs in your morning meal. This combination helps stabilize blood sugar, provides lasting energy, and keeps those pesky cravings at bay.

And here's a pro tip: try to eat your breakfast within an hour of waking up. This helps kickstart your metabolism and sets you up for a day of balanced eating.

So, rise and shine, beautiful! Your metabolism is waiting to be jumpstarted, and these delicious breakfasts are just the ticket. Who knew healthy eating could taste this good? Now, go forth and conquer your mornings like the metabolic confusion queen you are!

Alright, let's dive into the delicious world of lunch and dinner dishes that'll keep your metabolism on its toes! I'm excited to share some game-changing meal ideas that are not only tasty but also tailored to your endomorph body type. Get ready for a culinary adventure that'll transform your relationship with food and set you on the path to your ideal figure.

Chapter 7: Lunch and Dinner Dishes That Keep Your Body Guessing

Hey there, food lovers and health seekers! Welcome to the heart of our metabolic confusion journey - the main meals that'll make your taste buds dance and your body thrive. As an endomorph woman, you've got a unique relationship with food, and it's time we use that to your advantage. Let's turn those genes of yours from foes to friends, shall we?

The Magic of Metabolic Confusion on Your Plate

Before we jump into the recipes, let's chat about why these meals are your secret weapon. The metabolic confusion diet isn't about deprivation - it's about smart choices that keep your body guessing. By varying your calorie intake and macronutrient balance, you're essentially giving your metabolism a gentle nudge, saying, "Hey there, time to wake up and get to work!"

For us endomorphs, this approach is like striking gold. Our bodies are efficient at storing energy **(hello, stubborn fat!),** but with these meals, we're going to flip the script. We'll use protein to build lean muscle, complex carbs for sustained energy, and a rainbow of veggies to flood our systems with nutrients. The result? A body that burns more efficiently, even when you're Netflix and chilling.

Protein-Packed Main Courses: Your Metabolic Fuel

Alright, let's talk protein - the superstar macronutrient that's going to revolutionize your meals. For endomorphs, protein is like that friend who always has your back. It helps build lean muscle, keeps you feeling full, and even burns extra calories during digestion. But we're not talking about bland chicken breasts here - oh no, we're getting creative!

1. Zesty Lemon Herb Grilled Chicken: This dish is a flavor explosion that'll make your taste buds do a happy dance. The secret? A marinade of lemon juice, garlic, and a blend of fresh herbs. The acidity of the lemon actually helps tenderize the chicken, making it juicier and easier to digest. Plus, the vitamin C in the lemon boosts iron absorption from the chicken - talk about a power couple!

Prep time: 10 minutes (plus 2 hours marinating)
Cook time: 15 minutes
Ingredients:
- 4 boneless, skinless chicken breasts
- Juice of 2 lemons
- 2 cloves garlic, minced
- 1 tbsp each of fresh rosemary, thyme, and oregano, chopped
- 2 tbsp olive oil
- Salt and pepper to taste

Instructions:

1. Mix lemon juice, garlic, herbs, olive oil, salt, and pepper in a bowl.

2. Place chicken in a ziplock bag, pour in the marinade, and refrigerate for 2 hours.

3. Preheat grill to medium-high.

4. Grill chicken for 6-7 minutes per side, or until internal temperature reaches 165°F (74°C).

Nutritional value (per serving):

Calories: 220, Protein: 35g, Carbs: 2g, Fat: 8g

2. Mediterranean-Inspired Baked Cod

Fish is a fantastic protein source for endomorphs, and this dish brings the flavors of the Mediterranean right to your plate. The tomatoes and olives provide a dose of heart-healthy fats, while the fish offers lean protein that's easy on digestion.

Prep time: 15 minutes

Cook time: 20 minutes

Ingredients:

- 4 cod fillets (about 6 oz each)

- 1 pint cherry tomatoes, halved

- 1/4 cup Kalamata olives, pitted and chopped

- 2 tbsp capers

- 2 cloves garlic, minced

- 2 tbsp olive oil

- Juice of 1 lemon

- 1 tsp dried oregano

- Salt and pepper to taste

Instructions:

1. Preheat oven to 400°F (200°C).

2. In a bowl, mix tomatoes, olives, capers, garlic, 1 tbsp olive oil, and oregano.

3. Place cod fillets in a baking dish, drizzle with remaining oil and lemon juice.

4. Top with tomato mixture and bake for 15-20 minutes, until fish flakes easily.

Nutritional value (per serving):
Calories: 250, Protein: 30g, Carbs: 6g, Fat: 12g

Veggie-Loaded Sides: Color Your Plate, Boost Your Metabolism

Now, let's talk sides. As an endomorph, loading up on non-starchy veggies is like giving your metabolism a gentle nudge. They're low in calories but high in fiber, vitamins, and minerals. Plus, they add volume to your meals, helping you feel satisfied without overdoing it on calories.

1. Roasted Rainbow Vegetable Medley

This colorful side dish isn't just Instagram-worthy - it's a nutritional powerhouse. Each color represents different phytonutrients, so by eating the rainbow, you're giving your body a wide array of health benefits.

Prep time: 15 minutes
Cook time: 25 minutes
Ingredients:
- 1 red bell pepper, sliced
- 1 yellow bell pepper, sliced
- 1 small eggplant, cubed
- 1 zucchini, sliced
- 1 red onion, cut into wedges

- 2 tbsp olive oil

- 1 tsp dried thyme

- 1 tsp dried rosemary

- Salt and pepper to taste

- 1 tbsp balsamic vinegar (added after roasting)

Instructions:

1. Preheat oven to 425°F (220°C).

2. Toss vegetables with olive oil, herbs, salt, and pepper.

3. Spread on a baking sheet and roast for 20-25 minutes, stirring halfway through.

4. Drizzle with balsamic vinegar before serving.

Nutritional value (per serving):

Calories: 120, Protein: 3g, Carbs: 14g, Fat: 7g

2. Cauliflower "Mac" and Cheese

Who says comfort food can't be healthy? This clever swap uses cauliflower instead of pasta, dramatically reducing the carb content while pumping up the nutrients.

Prep time: 10 minutes

Cook time: 25 minutes

Ingredients:

- 1 large head cauliflower, cut into florets
- 1 cup plain Greek yogurt
- 1 cup shredded cheddar cheese
- 1/4 cup grated Parmesan cheese
- 2 tbsp butter
- 1/4 tsp garlic powder
- Salt and pepper to taste
- 2 tbsp chopped chives for garnish

Instructions:

1. Steam cauliflower until tender, about 10 minutes.

2. In a saucepan, melt butter and stir in Greek yogurt, cheddar, Parmesan, and garlic powder.

3. Add steamed cauliflower to the cheese sauce and stir gently to coat.

4. Transfer to a baking dish, top with extra cheese if desired, and broil for 3-5 minutes until golden.

5. Garnish with chives before serving.

Nutritional value (per serving):
Calories: 180, Protein: 14g, Carbs: 8g, Fat: 12g

One-Pot Wonders: Because You've Got Better Things to Do Than Dishes

Life gets hectic, but that's no excuse to let your nutrition slide. These one-pot meals are your secret weapon for busy days. They're easy to make, packed with nutrients, and best of all - **minimal cleanup required!**

1. Metabolic Confusion Chicken and Vegetable Soup

This soup is like a warm hug for your metabolism. The combination of lean protein, fiber-rich vegetables, and a secret ingredient - apple cider vinegar - makes it a powerhouse meal that's as comforting as it is nutritious.

Prep time: 15 minutes
Cook time: 30 minutes

Ingredients:

- 1 lb boneless, skinless chicken breast, cubed
- 1 onion, diced
- 2 carrots, sliced

- 2 celery stalks, sliced

- 1 zucchini, diced

- 1 can diced tomatoes

- 6 cups low-sodium chicken broth

- 2 tbsp apple cider vinegar

- 1 tsp dried thyme

- 1 tsp dried rosemary

- 2 cups baby spinach

- Salt and pepper to taste

Instructions:

1. In a large pot, sauté onion, carrots, and celery until softened.

2. Add chicken and cook until no longer pink.

3. Add remaining ingredients except spinach. Simmer for 20 minutes.

4. Stir in spinach and cook for an additional 2 minutes.

Nutritional value (per serving):

Calories: 200, Protein: 25g, Carbs: 15g, Fat: 5g

2. Spicy Turkey and Sweet Potato Skillet

This skillet meal is the perfect balance of lean protein, complex carbs, and vegetables. The addition of cinnamon isn't just for flavor - it may help regulate blood sugar levels, which is especially beneficial for endomorphs.

Prep time: 10 minutes
Cook time: 25 minutes

Ingredients:

- 1 lb lean ground turkey
- 2 medium sweet potatoes, diced
- 1 red bell pepper, diced

- 1 onion, diced

- 2 cloves garlic, minced

- 1 can black beans, drained and rinsed

- 1 tsp ground cumin

- 1 tsp smoked paprika

- 1/2 tsp cinnamon

- 1/4 tsp cayenne pepper (adjust to taste)

- Salt and pepper to taste

- 2 cups baby spinach

- Fresh cilantro for garnish

Instructions:

1. In a large skillet, brown the turkey over medium heat.

2. Add sweet potatoes, bell pepper, onion, and garlic. Cook until vegetables are tender.

3. Stir in black beans and spices. Cook for an additional 5 minutes.

4. Add spinach and cook until wilted.

5. Garnish with cilantro before serving.

Nutritional value (per serving):

Calories: 350, Protein: 30g, Carbs: 35g, Fat: 10g

The Art of Meal Prepping for Success

Before we wrap up, let's talk strategy. Meal prepping isn't just for fitness influencers - it's a game-changer for busy endomorphs like yourself. Spend a couple of hours on the weekend prepping proteins, chopping veggies, and portioning out snacks. Future you will be so grateful when you can throw together a balanced meal in minutes on a hectic weeknight.

Try this simple meal prep routine:

1. Grill a batch of Zesty Lemon Herb Chicken

2. Roast a big tray of Rainbow Vegetables

3. Make a pot of Metabolic Confusion Soup

With these components ready to go, you can mix and match throughout the week, ensuring you always have a balanced, metabolism-boosting meal at your fingertips.

Remember, the key to the metabolic confusion approach is variety. Don't be afraid to experiment with these recipes, swapping ingredients or trying new spice combinations. Your body (and taste buds) will thank you for keeping things interesting!

In Conclusion: Your Plate, Your Power

There you have it, folks - a treasure trove of lunch and dinner ideas that are tasty, nutritious, and perfectly tailored for your endomorph body type. These meals are more than just fuel - they're your secret weapon in outsmarting your genes and achieving that ideal figure.

By focusing on protein-packed main courses, loading up on veggie-rich sides, and embracing the convenience of one-pot meals, you're setting yourself up for success. You're not just eating - you're nourishing your body, boosting your metabolism, and taking control of your health journey.

Remember, this is about progress, not perfection. Some days you'll nail it, other days might be a bit off track - **and that's okay!** The beauty of the metabolic confusion approach is its flexibility. Keep your body guessing, enjoy your food, and watch as your energy soars and your body transforms.

So, who's ready to hit the kitchen and start this delicious adventure? Your ideal figure is waiting - let's go get it, one mouthwatering meal at a time!

Chapter 8

Smart Snacking for Endomorphs

Hey there, snack enthusiasts! Welcome to the chapter that's about to revolutionize your between-meal munching game. If you're an endomorph woman on a mission to outsmart your genes, you're in for a treat (pun totally intended). Let's dive into the world of smart snacking that'll keep you satisfied, energized, and on track to achieving your ideal figure.

Snacking Smarter, Not Harder

Listen up, because this is crucial: snacking isn't the enemy. In fact, for us endomorphs, strategic snacking can be a secret weapon in our metabolic arsenal. The key is choosing the right snacks at the right times. We're about to turn those mid-afternoon cravings and late-night munchies into opportunities for nourishing your body and boosting your metabolism.

Satisfying Between-Meal Bites

Let's kick things off with some snacks that'll keep you going strong between meals:

1. Greek Yogurt Parfait with a Twist

Forget boring old parfaits. We're jazzing things up with a protein-packed Greek yogurt base, topped with a sprinkle of cinnamon (hello, blood sugar regulation!), a handful of mixed berries, and a tablespoon of chopped nuts. The protein and healthy fats will keep you full, while the berries offer a sweet hit without spiking your blood sugar.

Quick recipe: Mix 1/2 cup Greek yogurt with 1/4 tsp cinnamon. Top with 1/4 cup mixed berries and 1 tbsp chopped almonds.

Nutrition: 150 calories, 15g protein, 12g carbs, 6g fat

2. Savory Roasted Chickpeas

These crunchy little guys are about to become your new best friend. Packed with fiber and protein, they'll satisfy that craving for something savory without derailing your progress. Plus, you can switch up the spices to keep things interesting.

Quick recipe: Drain and rinse a can of chickpeas, pat dry. Toss with 1 tbsp olive oil and your choice of spices (try smoked paprika, garlic powder, and a pinch of salt). Roast at 400°F for 20-30 minutes, shaking the pan halfway through.

Nutrition (per 1/4 cup serving): 120 calories, 5g protein, 15g carbs, 5g fat

3. Avocado Egg Salad on Cucumber Rounds

This snack is like a mini-meal that'll keep you satisfied for hours. The healthy fats from the avocado combined with the protein from the eggs make this a metabolic powerhouse.

Quick recipe: Mash 1/2 avocado with 1 chopped hard-boiled egg, a squeeze of lemon juice, and a dash of salt and pepper. Spread on cucumber slices for a refreshing crunch.

Nutrition: 200 calories, 10g protein, 8g carbs, 16g healthy fats

Pre and Post-Workout Fuel

Now, let's talk about fueling your workouts. As an endomorph, you need snacks that'll give you energy without weighing you down:

1. Pre-Workout Energy Balls: These little powerhouses are perfect for grabbing on your way to the gym. They're packed with complex carbs for sustained energy and a touch of protein to prime your muscles.

Quick recipe: Mix 1/2 cup rolled oats, 2 tbsp almond butter, 1 tbsp honey, and 1 tbsp chia seeds. Roll into balls and refrigerate.

Nutrition (per ball): 80 calories, 3g protein, 10g carbs, 4g fat

2. Post-Workout Protein Shake with a Twist

After your workout, your muscles are crying out for protein. This shake delivers, with a special ingredient to help fight inflammation.

Quick recipe: Blend 1 scoop vanilla protein powder, 1 cup unsweetened almond milk, 1/2

frozen banana, 1/2 cup frozen cauliflower (trust me on this!), and 1/4 tsp turmeric.

Nutrition: 220 calories, 25g protein, 20g carbs, 5g fat

Late-Night Craving Crushers

Ah, the dreaded late-night cravings. Instead of fighting them, let's satisfy them in a way that aligns with our goals:

1. Frozen Yogurt Bark

This treat feels indulgent but won't derail your progress. The protein in the yogurt helps stabilize blood sugar, while the dark chocolate offers antioxidants and a touch of sweetness.

Quick recipe: Spread 2 cups Greek yogurt on a parchment-lined baking sheet. Swirl in 2 tbsp honey and top with a handful of mixed berries and

1 oz chopped dark chocolate. Freeze until solid, then break into pieces.

Nutrition (per piece): 70 calories, 5g protein, 8g carbs, 3g fat

2. Spiced Pumpkin Seed Mix

Sometimes you just need something crunchy. This mix satisfies that craving while delivering a dose of minerals and healthy fats.

Quick recipe: Toss 1/4 cup pumpkin seeds with 1/4 tsp olive oil, a pinch of cinnamon, and a tiny dash of cayenne. Toast in a dry skillet until fragrant.

Nutrition: 160 calories, 7g protein, 4g carbs, 14g healthy fats

3. Warm Cinnamon Apple Slices; When you're craving something sweet and comforting, this snack hits the spot without added sugars.

Quick recipe: Slice an apple and microwave with a sprinkle of cinnamon and a tablespoon of water for 1-2 minutes. Top with 1 tbsp Greek yogurt for added protein.

Nutrition: 100 calories, 3g protein, 22g carbs, 0g fat

The Art of Mindful Snacking

Before we wrap up, let's chat about mindful snacking. It's not just about what you eat, but how you eat it. **Try these tips:**

1. Portion out your snacks instead of eating from the bag.

2. Sit down and really savor your snack - no mindless munching in front of the TV!

3. Ask yourself if you're truly hungry or just bored/stressed/tired.

4. Stay hydrated - sometimes thirst masquerades as hunger.

Remember, snacking is your friend on this journey. These options are designed to keep your metabolism humming, your energy levels stable, and your taste buds happy. Mix and match, get creative, and most importantly - enjoy! Your body will thank you for fueling it with these nutrient-dense, delicious snacks.

So, next time those cravings hit, you've got an arsenal of smart snacking options at your fingertips. Who said eating for your endomorph body type had to be boring? Now go forth and snack like the metabolic mastermind you are!

Chapter 9: Sweet Treats That Won't Derail Your Progress

Hey there, sweet tooth! Yes, I'm talking to you - the one who's been eyeing that chocolate bar in the pantry. Don't worry, I've got your back. Welcome to the chapter that's about to change your dessert game forever. We're diving into the world of guilt-free goodies that'll satisfy your cravings without sabotaging your progress. So buckle up, buttercup - it's time to indulge smartly!

Guilt-Free Desserts: Having Your Cake and Eating It Too

1. Chocolate Avocado Mousse

Who says chocolate can't be healthy? This creamy, dreamy mousse is about to blow your mind. The secret ingredient? Avocado! I know, I know - it sounds weird, but trust me on this one.

Here's the scoop: avocados are packed with healthy fats that'll keep you feeling full and satisfied. Plus, they give this mousse an incredibly silky texture without any added sugar. We're talking chocolate indulgence that actually loves you back!

Quick recipe: In a food processor, blend 2 ripe avocados, 1/4 cup unsweetened cocoa powder, 1/4 cup honey (or maple syrup for vegans), 1 tsp vanilla extract, and a pinch of salt until smooth. Chill for at least an hour before serving.

Nutritional breakdown (per serving): 150 calories, 3g protein, 15g carbs (5g fiber), 10g healthy fats

Pro tip: Top with a sprinkle of cacao nibs for some crunch and extra antioxidants!

2. Berry Chia Pudding

Calling all texture lovers! This pudding is like a party in your mouth. Chia seeds are the real MVPs here - they're loaded with omega-3 fatty acids, fiber, and protein. When soaked, they plump up into a tapioca-like consistency that's utterly addictive.

The best part? You can prep this the night before and wake up to a breakfast that tastes like dessert. Talk about starting your day on a sweet note!

Quick recipe: Mix 1/4 cup chia seeds with 1 cup unsweetened almond milk, 1 tsp vanilla extract, and 1 tbsp honey. Let it sit overnight in the fridge. **In the morning,** top with a handful of mixed berries and a sprinkle of sliced almonds.

Nutritional breakdown (per serving): 220 calories, 8g protein, 25g carbs (13g fiber), 12g healthy fats

Smoothies and Shakes: Sip Your Way to Satisfaction

3. Green Goddess Protein Smoothie

Don't let the color fool you - this smoothie is a dessert in disguise. It's packed with spinach (I promise you can't taste it) for a nutrient boost, but the star of the show is the banana and vanilla protein powder combo that makes it taste like a milkshake.

This is your go-to when you're craving something sweet but also want to nourish your body. It's like giving your cells a big, delicious hug.

Quick recipe: Blend 1 cup unsweetened almond milk, 1 frozen banana, 1 cup spinach, 1 scoop vanilla protein powder, 1 tbsp almond butter, and a handful of ice until smooth.

Nutritional breakdown: 300 calories, 25g protein, 30g carbs, 10g healthy fats

4. Chocolate Cherry "Nice" Cream

Who needs ice cream when you can have "nice" cream? This frozen treat is made with frozen bananas as a base, giving it that creamy texture you crave without any added sugars or dairy.

The combination of chocolate and cherries is like a Black Forest cake in a bowl, minus the guilt. Plus, cherries are natural sources of melatonin, making this a perfect evening treat to satisfy your sweet tooth and potentially help you sleep better. Win-win!

Quick recipe: In a food processor, blend 2 frozen bananas, 1/2 cup frozen cherries, 2 tbsp unsweetened cocoa powder, and a splash of almond milk until smooth and creamy.

Nutritional breakdown (per serving): 150 calories, 3g protein, 35g carbs, 1g fat

Baked Goods with a Healthy Twist: Because Sometimes You Need to Turn On the Oven

5. Almond Flour Chocolate Chip Cookies

Cookie monsters, rejoice! These little gems are about to become your new obsession. By swapping regular flour for almond flour, we're amping up the protein and healthy fats while keeping the carbs in check.

These cookies are chewy, gooey, and everything a good chocolate chip cookie should be. The best part? They won't send your blood sugar on a rollercoaster ride.

Quick recipe: Mix 2 cups almond flour, 1/4 cup melted coconut oil, 1/4 cup maple syrup, 1 egg, 1 tsp vanilla extract, 1/2 tsp baking soda, and a pinch of salt. Fold in 1/4 cup dark chocolate chips. Scoop onto a baking sheet and bake at 350°F for 12-15 minutes.

Nutritional breakdown (per cookie): 120 calories, 4g protein, 8g carbs, 9g healthy fats

6. Zucchini Brownie Bites

Brownies with veggies? Oh yes, we did! These fudgy bites are the perfect way to satisfy your chocolate cravings while sneaking in some extra nutrients. The zucchini adds moisture and fiber, while the cocoa powder brings that rich chocolate flavor you're after.

These are perfect for when you need a chocolate fix but don't want to go overboard. Plus, they're so good, you might just fool some veggie-haters in your life!

Quick recipe: Mix 1 cup grated zucchini (squeezed dry), 1 cup almond flour, 1/2 cup unsweetened cocoa powder, 1/4 cup honey, 2 eggs, 1/4 cup melted coconut oil, 1 tsp vanilla extract, 1/2 tsp baking soda, and a pinch of salt. Pour into a mini muffin tin and bake at 350°F for 15-18 minutes.

Nutritional breakdown (per brownie bite): 90 calories, 3g protein, 7g carbs, 7g healthy fats

The Sweet Secret to Success

Here's the deal, dessert lovers: it's all about balance and smart choices. These treats are designed to satisfy your sweet cravings without derailing your progress. They're packed with nutrients, lower in sugar, and full of flavor.

Remember, enjoying a treat now and then is part of a healthy, sustainable lifestyle. The key is to savor every bite mindfully. Really taste your food, enjoy the flavors and textures, and listen to your body's fullness cues.

And hey, if you happen to indulge in a "regular" dessert occasionally, don't sweat it! One treat won't make or break your progress. It's what you do consistently that counts.

So go ahead, whip up one of these goodies and enjoy it without an ounce of guilt. You're nourishing your body and soul, and that's something to celebrate. **Sweet dreams, dessert queens - you've got this!**

Chapter 10: Lifestyle Factors: Exercise, Sleep, and Stress Management

Hey there, lifestyle warriors! Welcome to the chapter that's about to revolutionize your whole approach to health. We're not just talking food here – we're diving into the trifecta of total well-being: exercise, sleep, and stress management. Buckle up, because this is where the magic happens for us endomorph women!

Workouts That Complement the Diet: Sweat Smart, Not Hard

Alright, let's kick things off with movement. As an endomorph, you've probably heard that you need to exercise like crazy to see results. Well, I'm here to flip that script. It's not about killing yourself in the gym – it's about moving in ways that complement your body type and diet. Let's break it down:

1. Strength Training: Your New Best Friend

Listen up, because this is crucial: lifting weights is your secret weapon. I know, I know – you might be worried about bulking up. But here's the truth: strength training will help you build lean muscle, boost your metabolism, and sculpt that figure you're after.

Try this: Start with 2-3 strength sessions per week. Focus on compound movements like squats, deadlifts, and push-ups. Don't be afraid to lift heavy – you're stronger than you think!

Pro tip: Keep a workout journal. Tracking your progress is incredibly motivating and helps you see how far you've come.

2. HIIT: The Time-Efficient Calorie Torcher High-Intensity Interval Training **(HIIT) is** like a cheat code for endomorphs. It burns calories during the workout and keeps your metabolism revved up for hours after. Plus, it's quick – perfect for busy schedules.

Give this a shot: Try a 20-minute HIIT workout. Do 30 seconds of all-out effort (think burpees, mountain climbers, or jump squats) followed by 30 seconds of rest. Repeat for 10 rounds. You'll be sweating and smiling in no time!

3. Low-Impact Cardio: The Unsung Hero

Don't discount the power of a good walk or swim. Low-impact cardio is great for recovery, stress relief, and burning fat without stressing your joints.

Challenge: Take a 30-minute walk after dinner each night. It'll aid digestion, help you unwind, and contribute to your overall calorie burn. Win-win-win!

The Importance of Quality Sleep: Beauty Rest Isn't Just a Saying

Okay, sleepyheads, this one's for you. Quality sleep is like a magic potion for endomorphs. It helps regulate hormones, reduces cravings, and supports muscle recovery. But it's not just about quantity – quality matters too.

Try these sleep-boosting tips:

1. Stick to a schedule: Try to go to bed and wake up at the same time every day, even on weekends. Your body will thank you!

2. Create a bedtime routine: Maybe it's a warm bath, some light stretching, or reading a book. Signal to your body that it's time to wind down.

3. Make your bedroom a sleep sanctuary: Keep it cool, dark, and quiet. Invest in comfortable bedding – you spend a third of your life in bed, after all!

4. Cut the screens: The blue light from phones and tablets can mess with your sleep hormones. Try to disconnect at least an hour before bed.

Sweet dreams challenge: This week, commit to 7-8 hours of quality sleep each night. Notice how it affects your energy, cravings, and overall mood.

Stress-Busting Techniques for Hormonal Balance: Zen and the Art of Endomorph Maintenance

Alright, let's talk stress. For us endomorphs, stress isn't just an emotional issue – it can seriously impact our hormones and make weight management tougher. But don't stress about stress (see what I did there?). We've got some tricks up our sleeves:

1. Mindful Meditation: Your New Superpower
I get it – the idea of sitting still and "doing nothing" might seem strange. But trust me, a few minutes of

mindfulness can work wonders for your stress levels and hormonal balance.

Start here: **Try the "5-5-5"** technique. Inhale for 5 counts, hold for 5, then exhale for 5. Repeat for 5 minutes. It's simple, but powerful.

2. Yoga: Flexibility for Body and Mind

Yoga is like a two-for-one deal: you get the benefits of movement and stress relief in one package. Plus, it's great for improving flexibility and body awareness.

Give it a go: Look up **"yoga for beginners"** on YouTube and try a **15-minute session**. Focus on how you feel during and after the practice.

3. Journaling: Brain Dump for Inner Peace

Sometimes, the best way to deal with stress is to get it out of your head and onto paper. Journaling can help you process emotions, identify patterns, and find solutions.

Try this: Spend **5 minutes** each night writing down three things you're grateful for and one thing you're looking forward to tomorrow.

4. Nature Therapy: The Great Outdoors is Calling

Never underestimate the power of fresh air and green spaces. Spending time in nature can lower stress hormones and boost your mood.

Weekend challenge: Find a local park or nature trail and spend at least 30 minutes exploring. Breathe deep and soak in the scenery.

Putting It All Together: Your Lifestyle Action Plan

Alright, superstar, you've got all the pieces – now let's put them together:

1. Movement: Aim for 3 strength training sessions, 2 HIIT workouts, and daily walks each week.

2. Sleep: Prioritize 7-8 hours of quality sleep per night. Stick to a consistent schedule.

3. Stress Management: Choose one stress-busting technique to practice daily, even if it's just for 5 minutes.

Remember, it's not about perfection – it's about progress. Small, consistent changes add up to big results over time. You've got this!

Final Thoughts: Embrace the Journey

Listen, amazing endomorph woman, you're on a journey to outsmart your genes and achieve your ideal figure. But here's the real secret: it's not just about the destination. It's about creating a lifestyle that makes you feel energized, balanced, and confident every single day.

So embrace the process. Celebrate the small victories. Be kind to yourself on the tough days. And remember – you're not just changing your body, you're transforming your life.

Now go out there and show the world what an endomorph woman can do! You've got the knowledge, the tools, and the power. **It's time to shine!**

Conclusion

Your Roadmap to Long-Term Success

Hey there, superstar! You've made it to the finish line - or should I say, the starting line of your new lifestyle? Welcome to the chapter that's going to tie everything together and set you up for long-lasting success. Grab a cup of tea (or your beverage of choice), get comfy, and let's chart your course for the amazing journey ahead!

Maintaining Results: Keeping the Momentum Going

Alright, let's address the elephant in the room - maintaining your results. You've put in the hard work, you're seeing changes, and now you're wondering, **"How do I keep this going?" Don't worry, I've got your back!**

1. The 80/20 Rule: Your New Best Friend

Here's the deal - striving for perfection is exhausting and, frankly, unnecessary. Enter the 80/20 rule. Aim to stick to your healthy habits 80% of the time, and allow yourself some flexibility for the other 20%. This isn't just about food - it applies to exercise, sleep, and stress management too.

Try this: Each week, plan out your meals and workouts. Make sure 80% align with what we've discussed in this book. For the other 20%, allow yourself to indulge a bit or take a rest day. It's all about balance, baby!

2. Regular Check-Ins: Your Personal Progress Report

You know how your car needs regular tune-ups? Well, so do you! Schedule regular check-ins with yourself to assess how you're doing and what might need tweaking.

Action step: Set a monthly date with yourself. Review your food diary, workout log, and how you're feeling overall. Celebrate your wins and identify areas for improvement.

3. Keep Learning: Knowledge is Power

The health and fitness world is always evolving, and so should you. Stay curious and keep expanding your knowledge.

Challenge: Each month, learn about one new aspect of health or nutrition. It could be a new recipe, a different workout style, or a meditation technique. Keep that beautiful brain of yours engaged!

Troubleshooting Common Challenges: Because Life Happens

Let's face it - life isn't always smooth sailing. But that doesn't mean you can't navigate the choppy waters. Here are some common challenges and how to tackle them:

1. Plateau Blues: When Progress Seems to Stall Hitting a plateau is normal, but it can be frustrating. If you feel stuck, it's time to shake things up.

Try this: Introduce a new type of workout, experiment with different recipes, or adjust your

macronutrient balance. Sometimes, a little change can jumpstart your progress.

2. Social Situations: Navigating Dining Out and Parties

Social events can be tricky, but they don't have to derail your progress.

Strategy: Before going out, have a small protein-rich snack. When you're there, focus on lean proteins and veggies, and allow yourself a small treat if you want. Remember, it's about enjoying life while staying on track.

3. Stress Overload: When Life Gets Crazy

We all have those periods when stress seems to take over. The key is not letting it sabotage your hard work.

Coping technique: When you feel overwhelmed, take a pause. Use the 5-5-5 breathing technique we discussed earlier. Remember, a few minutes of self-care can make a world of difference.

4. Motivation Dips: Rekindling Your Fire

It's normal for motivation to ebb and flow. When you're feeling less than inspired, it's time to reconnect with your 'why'.

Boost your mojo: Look back at your initial goals. How far have you come? What's still driving you? Sometimes, reminding yourself of your journey can reignite that spark.

Celebrating Non-Scale Victories: Because You're More Than a Number

Listen up, because this is important: your worth is not determined by a number on a scale. Let's talk about celebrating all the amazing non-scale victories you'll experience:

1. Energy Boost: Conquering Your Day Remember how you used to feel sluggish by mid-afternoon? Notice how you're now powering through your days with more pep in your step. That's worth celebrating!

2. Strength Gains: Embrace Your Inner Amazon Maybe you've graduated from knee push-ups to full push-ups, or you're lifting heavier weights. Heck, maybe you can now open that stubborn jar without help. You're getting stronger, and that's awesome!

3. Improved Sleep: Sweet Dreams Are Made of This

Are you falling asleep faster and waking up more refreshed? That's not just good luck - it's the result of your hard work.

4. Clothes Fitting Differently: Your Personal Fashion Show

Perhaps your favorite jeans are a bit looser, or you're feeling more confident in that dress you've had in the back of your closet. Strut your stuff, gorgeous!

5. Mood Boost: Happiness is the Best Accessory Notice how you're smiling more? Feeling more confident? That glow isn't just from your new

skincare routine - it's the result of taking care of yourself inside and out.

Celebration challenge: Each week, identify and celebrate at least one non-scale victory. Write it down, share it with a friend, or treat yourself to something special (maybe a new workout outfit or a relaxing bubble bath).

Your Roadmap to Success: The Journey Continues

As we wrap up this book, remember - this isn't the end. It's just the beginning of your amazing journey. You've got the knowledge, the tools, and most importantly, the power within you to achieve your goals.

Here's your roadmap to continued success:

1. Stay consistent with your healthy habits, but allow for flexibility.

2. Keep learning and adapting your approach as needed.

3. Face challenges head-on, knowing you have the strategies to overcome them.

4. Celebrate all your victories, big and small.

5. Above all, be kind to yourself. This journey is about progress, not perfection.

Final Thoughts: You've Got This!

Incredible endomorph woman, you are capable of amazing things. You've taken the first step by reading this book, and now it's time to put it all into action. Remember, every day is a new opportunity to make choices that align with your goals.

There will be ups and downs, triumphs and challenges. Embrace them all as part of your unique journey. You're not just changing your body - you're transforming your life.

So go out there and show the world what you're made of. You're strong, you're capable, and you're on your way to becoming the best version of yourself. I believe in you, and I hope you believe in yourself too.

Here's to your health, your happiness, and your success. You've got this, superstar!
Thank you for reading!If you found it enjoyable, please consider leaving a review. Your feedback helps others find the book and reach those who might benefit from it. Your support is deeply appreciated!